I0782759

BREAST CANCER SMOOTHIES FOR BEGINNERS

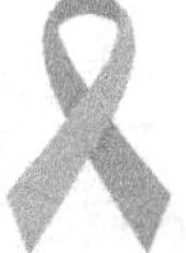

Delicious Recipes to Help During Cancer Treatment and Recovery

JANE BABB

Copyright © 2024 Jane Babb

All rights reserved. No part of this book may be reproduced in any form without written permission from the author. Any unauthorized copying, distribution, or use of this book or its contents, including but not limited to excerpts is strictly prohibited and may be a violation of copyright law.

Disclaimer:

The information contained in this book is based on the author's years of research and experience and it is intended for informational and educational purposes. It is not in any way meant to eliminate the need for consulting with a medical doctor.

The author and publisher make no warranties or representations, either express or implied, for the contents of this book, including but not limited to the implied warranties of merchantability and fitness for a particular purpose. The author and publisher shall not be liable for any damages or injuries arising from the use of this book.

TABLE OF CONTENTS

INTRODUCTION

Dear Reader,

I am delighted to embark on this journey with you as we explore the powerful synergy between wholesome ingredients and your well-being.

In the face of a breast cancer diagnosis, the significance of nutrition takes center stage. It is not just about what you eat; it is about the nurturing elixirs you sip, the vibrant colors you blend, and the energy you infuse into your body. This book is crafted with care and empathy, recognizing the challenges that come with the journey you are on.

The chapters ahead are designed to be your companion, offering guidance on creating delicious, nutrient-dense smoothies tailored to support you through each step of your breast cancer wellness path. From understanding the role of nutrition to providing a range of recipes and addressing common concerns, this book aims to empower you to make informed and enjoyable choices for your health.

Smoothies aren't just drinks; they are a celebration of life, a delicious way to embrace the healing power of nature's bounty. In breast cancer management, the significance of nutrition cannot be overstated. Cancer as a formidable adversary, not only challenges the body physically but also necessitates a holistic approach to support its healing. Nutrition plays a pivotal role in this holistic strategy, acting as a foundation for vitality and resilience.

Within the context of breast cancer, nutrition assumes multifaceted roles. It serves as a source of strength during treatments, aiding the body in tolerating the side effects of therapies such as chemotherapy and radiation. A well-nourished body is better equipped to combat fatigue, maintain muscle mass, and promote a swifter recovery.

Moreover, nutrition contributes to the prevention of malnutrition, a common concern during cancer treatment. Maintaining a balanced diet becomes paramount, ensuring the body receives the necessary nutrients for cellular repair and immune function. **This is where the concept of smoothies steps in, offering a delightful and efficient means to deliver a concentrated dose of essential nutrients.**

Smoothies, with their versatility and easy digestibility, become a palatable solution for individuals navigating the challenges of breast cancer. From antioxidants that combat oxidative stress to anti-inflammatory compounds that soothe the body, each ingredient in this book is carefully chosen to contribute to the overarching goal of supporting your health.

Each smoothie recipe in this book is for 1 serving.

CHAPTER 1: IMPORTANCE OF SMOOTHIES IN CANCER CARE

Smoothies hold a unique significance in the broader landscape of cancer wellness and these are some of the reasons why.

Easy Nutrient Absorption:

Smoothies, with their blended consistency, provide a gentle way for the body to absorb essential nutrients. This is particularly crucial in cancer care, where treatments may impact appetite and the ability to eat solid foods. The liquefied form of smoothies facilitates nutrient absorption, ensuring that the body receives the vital elements it needs for recovery.

Hydration Reinforcement:

Staying hydrated is paramount during cancer treatments, and smoothies offer a delicious way to meet this requirement. With a base of hydrating ingredients like fruits, vegetables, and liquids such as coconut water, smoothies become a tasty vehicle for replenishing fluids and maintaining optimal hydration levels.

Tailored Nutrition:

Each ingredient in a smoothie can be chosen intentionally to contribute to specific nutritional goals. Whether it's incorporating anti-inflammatory fruits or immune-boosting herbs, smoothies allow for a personalized approach to nutrition. This tailored aspect is particularly crucial in addressing the unique needs of individuals navigating breast cancer, where dietary considerations are paramount.

Caloric Density and Weight Maintenance:

For some undergoing cancer treatments, maintaining a healthy weight is a challenge. Smoothies, when crafted with nutrient-dense ingredients, offer a concentrated source of calories and nutrients. This can be especially beneficial in preventing unintended weight loss and supporting the body's energy needs during the healing process.

Taste and Texture Variety:

Cancer treatments can sometimes alter taste buds and make certain foods unappealing. Smoothies, with their wide array of flavors and textures, provide a versatile and enjoyable way to reintroduce variety into the diet. From sweet and fruity to creamy and nutty, there's a smoothie for every palate, making the culinary journey a more delightful one.

How This Book Can Help You

This book is crafted with the understanding that a breast cancer diagnosis is not just a medical event; it is a journey that touches every aspect of your life. Here is how this book can be a guiding companion on that journey.

Empowering with Knowledge:

This book provides insights into the nutritional aspects of each ingredient, helping you make informed choices about what goes into your body. This knowledge becomes a powerful ally in your quest for wellness.

Practical Guidance for Beginners:

Navigating a new dietary landscape can be overwhelming, especially for those who are new to the world of smoothies. This book is designed with simplicity in mind, offering practical guidance on getting started.

Culinary Joy in Every Sip:

Healing doesn't have to be bland. The recipes within these pages are crafted not just for their nutritional value but for the joy they can bring to your palate. Each sip is an opportunity to indulge in flavors that uplift your spirits and make the culinary aspect of your journey a delightful one.

Adaptability to Your Preferences:

Everyone's taste and dietary preferences are unique. This book encourages experimentation, offering a variety of recipes that can be adapted to suit your individual needs. Whether you have dietary restrictions, allergies, or specific flavor preferences, there's a smoothie here for you.

Kitchen Essentials for Smoothie Making

Creating delicious and nutritious smoothies doesn't require a fully stocked kitchen; a few key essentials can turn your culinary space into a vibrant smoothie haven. Let's explore the essential tools and ingredients that will make your smoothie-making experience both enjoyable and efficient.

High-Quality Blender:

Invest in a good-quality blender. Whether it's a high-powered blender or a reliable countertop version, having a blender that can efficiently break down fruits, vegetables, and other ingredients is crucial for achieving a smooth and creamy texture in your smoothies.

Fresh and Frozen Ingredients:

The foundation of a great smoothie lies in the freshness of your ingredients. Stock your kitchen with a variety of fresh fruits and vegetables, and don't forget to keep some frozen options on hand. Frozen fruits not only add a refreshing chill to your smoothies but also contribute to a thicker consistency.

Liquid Bases:

Choose from a variety of liquid bases to tailor your smoothie to your taste and nutritional preferences. Almond milk, coconut water, yogurt, or even green tea can add depth and flavor to your creations. Experiment with different bases to find the combination that suits you best.

Nut Butter and Seeds:

Enhance the nutritional profile of your smoothies by incorporating nut butter like almond or peanut butter. Seeds such as chia seeds, flaxseeds, or hemp seeds are excellent sources of omega-3 fatty acids and can contribute to the overall health benefits of your smoothies.

Leafy Greens:

A handful of leafy greens can elevate the nutritional content of your smoothies. Spinach, kale, or swiss chard are mild-flavored options that blend well with fruits, adding essential vitamins and minerals to your concoction.

Sweeteners and Flavor Boosters:

While fruits contribute natural sweetness, you may choose to add a touch of honey, maple syrup, or agave nectar for extra flavor. Experiment with spices like cinnamon, ginger, or turmeric to enhance the taste and provide additional health benefits.

Ice Cubes:

For those who prefer a frostier consistency, keep ice cubes on hand. They not only add a refreshing chill to your smoothies but also contribute to the desired thickness.

Measuring Cups and Spoons:

Accurate measurements ensure the right balance of flavors and nutritional content. Keep measuring cups and spoons handy to create consistent and well-balanced smoothies every time.

Glassware or Portable Cups:

Presentation matters, and having a collection of appealing glasses or portable cups can enhance the overall experience of enjoying your smoothies. Choose vessels that make your sipping experience a pleasure.

Cleaning Supplies:

Having a reliable set of cleaning supplies, including a bottle brush for your blender, makes the post-smoothie process quick and easy.

CHAPTER 2: NUTRITIONAL FOUNDATION

Overview of Nutrients Beneficial for Breast Cancer Patients

It is crucial to understand the role of nutrients in supporting the health and well-being of individuals on the breast cancer journey. Let's explore the key nutrients that play a vital role in supporting breast cancer patients.

Antioxidants:

Antioxidants are superheroes in the world of nutrition, and they play a crucial role in the context of breast cancer. Found in abundance in fruits like berries, citrus fruits, and vegetables, antioxidants help combat oxidative stress. This stress arises from an imbalance between free radicals and antioxidants and is linked to various diseases, including cancer. The colorful array of berries and fruits in your smoothies brings a powerful antioxidant punch.

Vitamins and Minerals:

Essential vitamins and minerals contribute to overall health and can be particularly beneficial during cancer care. Vitamin C, found in citrus fruits, supports the immune system, while vitamin K in leafy greens aids in blood clotting and bone health. Minerals like potassium in bananas and magnesium in nuts and seeds play roles in maintaining electrolyte balance and supporting muscle function.

Fiber:

A diet rich in fiber is known for its digestive benefits, but it also plays a role in regulating blood sugar levels and supporting heart health. Fruits, vegetables, and seeds in these smoothies contribute valuable dietary fiber, promoting gut health and assisting in the management of side effects from cancer treatments.

Omega-3 Fatty Acids:

Omega-3 fatty acids, found in sources like chia seeds, flaxseeds, and walnuts, have anti-inflammatory properties. Inflammation is linked to cancer progression, and incorporating these healthy fats into your smoothies can contribute to an anti-inflammatory diet.

Protein:

Protein is crucial for tissue repair, immune function, and maintaining muscle mass, all of which are significant considerations during breast cancer care. Greek yogurt, nut butter, and seeds in your smoothies provide protein to support your body's healing and recovery processes.

Phytochemicals:

Phytochemicals are bioactive compounds found in plants that have been associated with various health benefits, including cancer prevention. The diversity of fruits, vegetables, and herbs in your smoothies introduces a spectrum of phytochemicals, each with its unique potential for promoting health and well-being.

Hydration:

Staying hydrated is crucial during cancer care, especially when dealing with potential side effects like nausea. Smoothies with a high water content, combined with hydrating bases like coconut water or green tea, cucumber, and watermelon contribute to overall fluid intake, supporting hydration and maintaining optimal fluid balance.

Digestive Enzymes:

Certain fruits, such as pineapple and papaya, contain digestive enzymes like bromelain and papain, which can aid in digestion. These enzymes may be particularly beneficial for individuals experiencing digestive issues as a result of cancer treatments.

Caloric Density:

For those experiencing weight loss or challenges with appetite, the caloric density of smoothies can be adjusted to provide a concentrated source of energy. Adding ingredients like nut butter, avocados, or full-fat yogurt can enhance caloric content without compromising nutritional value.

Adaptogens:

While not traditional nutrients, adaptogens like turmeric and ginger are often incorporated into smoothies for their potential to help the body adapt to stress. These ingredients may provide comfort and support during the challenging times associated with breast cancer.

Anti-Inflammatory Ingredients for Healing

In breast cancer where inflammation is intricately linked to the disease's progression and treatment side effects, incorporating these ingredients into your smoothies becomes a deliberate and empowering choice for your well-being.

Turmeric:

Turmeric is a golden-hued spice celebrated for its potent anti-inflammatory compound, curcumin. Research suggests that curcumin may help reduce inflammation and oxidative stress. Including turmeric in your smoothies adds not just warmth to the flavor but also a boost of potential healing properties.

Ginger:

Ginger, with its spicy and aromatic profile, contains bioactive compounds with anti-inflammatory and antioxidant effects. Known for its soothing properties, ginger can provide comfort to those experiencing nausea or digestive discomfort during breast cancer treatments.

Berries:

Berries, such as blueberries, strawberries, and raspberries, are not only delicious but also rich in antioxidants and anti-inflammatory compounds. The vibrant colors of these fruits indicate the presence of anthocyanins, which have been associated with anti-inflammatory effects.

Leafy Greens:

Spinach, kale, and other leafy greens are powerhouse ingredients in combating inflammation. Packed with vitamins, minerals, and phytochemicals, these greens offer a nutritional punch that supports overall health and wellness.

Pineapple:

Pineapple contains bromelain, an enzyme known for its anti-inflammatory and digestive benefits. Including pineapple in your smoothies adds a tropical sweetness while contributing potential healing properties to the mix.

Avocado:

Creamy and nutrient-dense, avocados contain monounsaturated fats and antioxidants that may help reduce inflammation. Their velvety texture enhances the smoothness of your blend, offering a nourishing component to your healing journey.

Nuts and Seeds:

Almonds, walnuts, flaxseeds, and chia seeds are rich sources of omega-3 fatty acids and antioxidants. These ingredients contribute to an anti-inflammatory diet, supporting your body's resilience during breast cancer care.

Green Tea:

Green tea is a hydrating and antioxidant-rich base for your smoothies. The presence of catechins, a type of polyphenol, in green tea has been linked to anti-inflammatory effects, making it a wholesome addition to your healing concoctions.

Cinnamon:

Beyond its aromatic and comforting flavor, cinnamon harbors anti-inflammatory and antioxidant properties. Sprinkle a dash of cinnamon into your smoothies for both a delightful taste and potential health benefits.

Broccoli Sprouts:

Broccoli sprouts contain sulforaphane, a compound with anti-inflammatory and antioxidant effects. While small in size, these sprouts can add a nutritional punch to your smoothies, supporting your body's natural defence mechanisms.

Superfoods to Boost Immunity

In recognizing the unique challenges faced by individuals on the breast cancer journey, the incorporation of these immune-boosting superfoods into your smoothies will help during treatment and the recovery process.

Acai Berries:

Acai berries, rich in antioxidants, contribute to immune support by combating oxidative stress. Their deep purple hue signifies the presence of anthocyanins, which may have anti-inflammatory effects. Including acai berries in your smoothies adds not just a burst of color but a potential boost to your immune system.

Goji Berries:

Often referred to as a "superfruit," goji berries are packed with vitamins, minerals, and antioxidants. They contain beta-carotene, vitamin C, and other compounds that may support immune function.

Chia Seeds:

Chia seeds contain a lot of antioxidants, fiber, and omega-3 fatty acids. The combination of these nutrients supports overall health, including immune function. The gel-like consistency they develop when soaked adds a unique texture to your smoothies.

Spinach:

Leafy greens, such as spinach, are dense with vitamins, minerals, and phytochemicals. In particular, spinach is a great source of vitamin C and beta-carotene, both of which contribute to immune health.

Moringa Powder:

Moringa is rich in minerals, antioxidants, and vitamins. Its potential immune-boosting properties make moringa powder a valuable addition to your smoothies. It adds a mild, earthy flavor while infusing your blend with nutritional benefits.

Kiwi:

Kiwi is rich in vitamin C, providing more vitamin C per serving than many citrus fruits. Vitamin C is essential for immune function, and the sweet and tangy taste of kiwi makes it a delightful addition to your immune-boosting smoothies.

Spirulina:

Spirulina is a nutrient-dense blue-green algae that boasts a high protein content, essential vitamins, and minerals. Its potential immune-modulating effects make it a noteworthy superfood for those seeking to fortify their defences. A small amount of spirulina can add a vibrant green hue to your smoothies.

Turmeric:

Beyond its anti-inflammatory properties, turmeric contains curcumin, a compound that may enhance immune function. The earthy and slightly bitter flavor of turmeric adds depth to your smoothies while potentially providing immune support.

Cranberries:

Cranberries are known for their rich content of antioxidants, including vitamin C. They also contain compounds that may have antibacterial properties. The tart flavor of cranberries can be balanced with sweeter fruits in your smoothies, creating a harmonious blend of flavors.

Yogurt with Probiotics:

Yogurt with live and active cultures introduces probiotics, beneficial bacteria that support gut health. Since a significant portion of the immune system resides in the gut, maintaining a healthy balance of gut bacteria can contribute to overall immune function. Choose yogurt with probiotics to add a creamy and probiotic-rich element to your smoothies.

CHAPTER 3: FRUIT SMOOTHIES RECIPES

The recipes in this chapter feature a diverse range of fruits, each selected for its unique contribution to overall health and well-being. From the hydrating qualities of watermelon to the antioxidant-rich blueberries and the tropical sweetness of pineapple, these smoothies aim to bring joy to the palate while offering a nutritional boost.

We delve into the specifics of ingredients, preparation methods, and nutritional information for each recipe, ensuring that these smoothies are not only delicious but also tailored to support your needs as you undergo breast cancer treatment and recovery.

We understand that embracing a new dietary routine during treatment can be daunting, so we have kept these recipes refreshingly simple.

The focus is on accessible ingredients, easy preparation methods, and most importantly, on creating a pleasurable experience for you.

Berry Blast Smoothie

INGREDIENTS

1/2 cup blueberries (fresh or frozen)

1/2 cup strawberries, hulled (fresh or frozen)

1/4 cup raspberries (fresh or frozen)

1/4 cup blackberries (fresh or frozen)

1/2 banana

1/2 cup Greek yogurt

1/2 cup almond milk

1 tablespoon chia seeds

1 teaspoon honey (optional)

Ice cubes (optional)

PREPARATION

In a blender, combine blueberries, strawberries, raspberries, blackberries, bananas, Greek yogurt, almond milk, and chia seeds.

If desired, add a teaspoon of honey for sweetness.

Blend on high speed until a smooth and creamy texture is achieved.

If a colder consistency is preferred, add ice cubes and blend again until well incorporated.

Pour the smoothie into a glass and garnish with a few whole berries.

NUTRITIONAL INFORMATION

Calories: 250 kcal, Protein: 12g

Fiber: 10g, Fat: 5g

Carbohydrates: 40g

Citrus Sunshine Smoothie

INGREDIENTS

1/2 cup orange segments (fresh)

1/2 cup grapefruit segments (fresh)

1/2 cup pineapple chunks (fresh or frozen)

1/2 banana

1/2 cup Greek yogurt

1/2 cup coconut water

1 tablespoon flaxseeds

1 teaspoon turmeric powder

1 teaspoon honey (optional)

Ice cubes (optional)

PREPARATION

In a blender, combine orange segments, grapefruit segments, pineapple chunks, banana, Greek yogurt, coconut water, flaxseeds, and turmeric powder.

If desired, add a teaspoon of honey for sweetness.

Blend on high speed until the mixture is smooth.

If a colder consistency is preferred, add ice cubes and blend again until well incorporated.

Pour into a glass.

Garnish with a slice of citrus or a sprinkle of turmeric

NUTRITIONAL INFORMATION

Calories: 280 kcal, Protein: 11g

Fiber: 8g, Fat: 6g

Carbohydrates: 45g

Mango Antioxidant Blend Smoothie

INGREDIENTS

1 cup mango
chunks (fresh or
frozen)

1/2 cup
strawberries,
hulled (fresh or
frozen)

1/2 cup
blueberries (fresh
or frozen)

1/2 banana

1/2 cup plain
Greek yogurt

1/2 cup almond
milk

1 tablespoon chia
seeds

1 teaspoon honey
(optional)

Ice cubes
(optional)

PREPARATION

In a blender, combine mango chunks, strawberries, blueberries, banana, Greek yogurt, almond milk, and chia seeds.

If desired, add a teaspoon of honey for sweetness.

Blend on high speed until the mixture is velvety smooth.

For a cooler temperature, add ice cubes and blend again until well incorporated.

Pour into a glass.

Garnish with a slice of mango or a few whole berries.

NUTRITIONAL INFORMATION

Calories: 280 kcal, Protein: 12g

Fiber: 8g, Fat: 5g

Carbohydrates: 45g

Tropical Oasis Smoothie

INGREDIENTS

1/2 cup pineapple chunks (fresh or frozen)

1/2 cup mango chunks (fresh or frozen)

1/2 banana

1/2 cup coconut milk

1/2 cup orange juice (freshly squeezed)

1 tablespoon flaxseeds

1 teaspoon turmeric powder

1 teaspoon honey (optional)

Ice cubes (optiona

PREPARATION

In a blender, combine pineapple chunks, mango chunks, banana, coconut milk, freshly squeezed orange juice, flaxseeds, and turmeric powder.

If desired, add a teaspoon of honey for sweetness.

Blend on high speed until the mixture achieves a smooth consistency.

For a refreshing chill, incorporate ice cubes and blend again.

Pour into a glass. Garnish with a slice of pineapple or a sprinkle of turmeric.

NUTRITIONAL INFORMATION

Calories: 290 kcal, Protein: 5g

Fiber: 7g, Fat: 12g

Carbohydrates: 45g

Citrus Sunrise Smoothie

INGREDIENTS

1/2 cup orange segments (fresh)

1/2 cup grapefruit segments (fresh)

1/2 banana

1/2 cup Greek yogurt

1/2 cup almond milk

1 tablespoon chia seeds

1 teaspoon honey (optional)

Ice cubes (optional

PREPARATION

In a blender, combine fresh orange segments, grapefruit segments, banana, Greek yogurt, almond milk, and chia seeds.

Add a teaspoon of honey for a touch of sweetness if preferred.

Blend the mixture on high speed until it reaches a smooth consistency.

For a cooler temperature, add ice cubes and blend again until well incorporated.

Pour into a glass.

Optional: Garnish with a slice of citrus or a sprinkle of chia seeds.

NUTRITIONAL INFORMATION

Calories: 250 kcal, Protein: 11g

Fiber: 8g, Fat: 6g

Carbohydrates: 40g

Pomegranate Power Punch Smoothie

INGREDIENTS

1/2 cup pomegranate arils

1/2 cup berries mix (blueberries, raspberries, strawberries)

1/2 banana

1/2 cup plain Greek yogurt

1/2 cup pomegranate juice (100% pure)

1 tablespoon hemp seeds

1 teaspoon honey (optional)

Ice cubes (optional)

PREPARATION

In a blender, combine pomegranate arils, mixed berries, banana, plain Greek yogurt, pomegranate juice, and hemp seeds.

Add a teaspoon of honey for a touch of sweetness if preferred.

Blend the mixture on high speed.

For a cooler consistency, include ice cubes and blend again until well incorporated.

Pour the antioxidant-rich smoothie into a glass.

Optional: Garnish with a few extra pomegranate arils or a sprinkle of hemp seeds.

NUTRITIONAL INFORMATION

Calories: 280 kcal, Protein: 12g

Fiber: 8g, Fat: 5g

Carbohydrates: 45g

Kiwi Berry Smoothie

INGREDIENTS

2 kiwis, peeled and sliced

1/2 cup mixed berries (strawberries, blueberries, raspberries)

1/2 banana

1/2 cup Greek yogurt

1/2 cup almond milk

1 tablespoon chia seeds

1 teaspoon honey (optional)

Ice cubes (optional)

PREPARATION

In a blender, combine sliced kiwis, mixed berries, banana, Greek yogurt, almond milk, and chia seeds.

Add a teaspoon of honey for a touch of sweetness if preferred.

Blend the mixture on high speed.

For a refreshing chill, include ice cubes and blend again until well incorporated.

Pour the nutrient-rich smoothie into a glass.

Optional: Garnish with a slice of kiwi or a few whole berries.

NUTRITIONAL INFORMATION

Calories: 250 kcal, Protein: 11g

Fiber: 8g, Fat: 5g

Carbohydrates: 40g

Fig Fusion Smoothie

INGREDIENTS

2 fresh figs, stems removed and halved

1/2 banana

1/2 cup pineapple chunks (fresh or frozen)

1/2 cup Greek yogurt

1/2 cup almond milk

1 tablespoon hemp seeds

1 teaspoon honey (optional)

Ice cubes (optional))

PREPARATION

In a blender, combine fresh figs, banana, pineapple chunks, Greek yogurt, almond milk, and hemp seeds.

Add a teaspoon of honey for a touch of sweetness if preferred.

Blend the mixture on high speed.

For a cooler consistency, add ice cubes and blend again until well combined.

Pour the smoothie into a glass.

Optional: Garnish with a fig slice or a sprinkle of hemp seeds.

NUTRITIONAL INFORMATION

Calories: 280 kcal, Protein: 12g

Fiber: 8g, Fat: 6g

Carbohydrates: 45g

Strawberry Serenity Smoothie

INGREDIENTS

1 cup strawberries, hulled (fresh or frozen)

1/2 cup banana

1/2 cup cucumber, peeled and chopped

1/2 cup plain Greek yogurt

1/2 cup almond milk

1 tablespoon flaxseeds

1 teaspoon honey (optional)

Ice cubes (optional)

PREPARATION

In a blender, combine strawberries, banana, cucumber, plain Greek yogurt, almond milk, and flaxseeds.

Add a teaspoon of honey for a touch of sweetness if preferred.

Blend the mixture on high speed.

For a cooler consistency, add ice cubes and blend again until well combined.

Pour the soothing smoothie into a glass.

Optional: Garnish with a strawberry slice or a drizzle of honey.

NUTRITIONAL INFORMATION

Calories: 250 kcal, Protein: 11g

Fiber: 8g, Fat: 6g

Carbohydrates: 40g

Pineapple Mint Smoothie

INGREDIENTS

1/2 cup pineapple chunks (fresh or frozen)

1/2 banana

1/2 cup cucumber, peeled and chopped

1/2 cup fresh mint leaves

1/2 cup Greek yogurt

1/2 cup coconut water

1 tablespoon chia seeds

1 teaspoon honey (optional)

Ice cubes (optional)

PREPARATION

In a blender, combine pineapple chunks, banana, cucumber, fresh mint leaves, Greek yogurt, coconut water, and chia seeds.

Add a teaspoon of honey for a touch of sweetness if preferred.

Blend the mixture on high speed.

For an extra chill, include ice cubes and blend again until well combined.

Pour the smoothie into a glass.

Optional: Garnish with a sprig of fresh mint or a slice of pineapple.

NUTRITIONAL INFORMATION

Calories: 240 kcal, Protein: 10g

Fiber: 6g, Fat: 5g

Carbohydrates: 40g

Grapes of Gratitude Smoothie

INGREDIENTS

1 cup red or green grapes, stems removed

1/2 cup pineapple chunks (fresh or frozen)

1/2 banana

1/2 cup plain Greek yogurt

1/2 cup coconut water

1 tablespoon hemp seeds

1 teaspoon honey (optional)

Ice cubes (optional)

PREPARATION

In a blender, combine red or green grapes, pineapple chunks, banana, plain Greek yogurt, coconut water, and hemp seeds.

Add a teaspoon of honey for a touch of sweetness if preferred.

Blend the mixture on high speed.

For an extra chill, include ice cubes and blend again until well combined.

Pour into a glass.

Optional: Garnish with a grape or a sprinkle of hemp seeds.

NUTRITIONAL INFORMATION

Calories: 250 kcal, Protein: 10g

Fiber: 5g, Fat: 6g

Carbohydrates: 40g

Blueberry Basil Bliss Smoothie

INGREDIENTS

1/2 cup blueberries (fresh or frozen)

1/2 cup strawberries, hulled (fresh or frozen)

1/2 banana

1/2 cup plain Greek yogurt

1/2 cup almond milk

1/4 cup fresh basil leaves

1 tablespoon chia seeds

1 teaspoon honey (optional)

Ice cubes (optional)

PREPARATION

In a blender, combine blueberries, strawberries, banana, plain Greek yogurt, almond milk, fresh basil leaves, and chia seeds.

Add a teaspoon of honey for a touch of sweetness if preferred.

Blend the mixture on high speed.

For a cooler consistency, add ice cubes and blend again until well combined.

Pour the vibrant smoothie into a glass.

Optional: Garnish with a basil leaf or a few extra blueberries.

NUTRITIONAL INFORMATION

Calories: 250 kcal, Protein: 12g

Fiber: 8g, Fat: 5g

Carbohydrates: 40g

Papaya Paradise Smoothie

INGREDIENTS

1 cup fresh papaya chunks, seeds removed

1/2 cup pineapple chunks (fresh or frozen)

1/2 banana

1/2 cup Greek yogurt

1/2 cup coconut milk

1 tablespoon flaxseeds

1 teaspoon honey (optional)

Ice cubes (optional)

PREPARATION

In a blender, combine fresh papaya chunks, pineapple chunks, banana, Greek yogurt, coconut milk, and flaxseeds.

Add a teaspoon of honey for a touch of sweetness if preferred.

Blend the mixture on high speed.

For a cooler consistency, add ice cubes and blend again until well combined.

Pour into a glass.

Optional: Garnish with a slice of papaya or a drizzle of honey.

NUTRITIONAL INFORMATION

Calories: 280 kcal, Protein: 11g

Fiber: 8g, Fat: 6g

Carbohydrates: 45g

Watermelon Wonder Smoothie

INGREDIENTS

1 cup fresh watermelon cubes, seeds removed

1/2 cup strawberries, hulled (fresh or frozen)

1/2 cup cucumber, peeled and chopped

1/2 banana

1/2 cup Greek yogurt

1/2 cup coconut water

1 tablespoon mint leaves

1 teaspoon chia seeds

1 teaspoon honey (optional)

Ice cubes (optional)

PREPARATION

In a blender, combine fresh watermelon cubes, strawberries, cucumber, banana, Greek yogurt, coconut water, mint leaves, and chia seeds.

Add a teaspoon of honey for a touch of sweetness if preferred.

Blend the mixture on high speed.

For an extra chill, include ice cubes and blend again until well combined.

Pour the hydrating smoothie into a glass.

Optional: Garnish with a mint sprig or a slice of watermelon.

NUTRITIONAL INFORMATION

Calories: 230 kcal, Protein: 9g

Fiber: 5g, Fat: 5g

Carbohydrates: 40g

Apple Infusion Smoothie

INGREDIENTS

1 medium-sized apple, cored and chopped

1/2 banana

1/2 cup rolled oats

1/2 cup plain Greek yogurt

1/2 cup almond milk

1/2 teaspoon ground cinnamon

1/4 teaspoon nutmeg

1 tablespoon flaxseeds

1 teaspoon honey (optional)

Ice cubes (optional)

PREPARATION

In a blender, combine chopped apple, banana, rolled oats, plain Greek yogurt, almond milk, ground cinnamon, nutmeg, and flaxseeds.

Add a teaspoon of honey for a touch of sweetness if preferred.

Blend the mixture on high speed.

For a colder consistency, include ice cubes and blend again until well incorporated.

Pour the nutritious smoothie into a glass.

Optional: Sprinkle a pinch of cinnamon on top.

NUTRITIONAL INFORMATION

Calories: 300 kcal, Protein: 12g

Fiber: 8g, Fat: 7g

Carbohydrates: 50g

Cherry Berry Smoothie

INGREDIENTS

1/2 cup cherries, pitted

1/2 cup mixed berries (blueberries, raspberries, strawberries)

1/2 banana

1/2 cup plain Greek yogurt

1/2 cup almond milk

1 tablespoon chia seeds

1 teaspoon honey (optional)

Ice cubes (optional)

PREPARATION

In a blender, combine pitted cherries, mixed berries, banana, plain Greek yogurt, almond milk, and chia seeds.

Add a teaspoon of honey for a touch of sweetness if preferred.

Blend the mixture on high speed.

For a cooler consistency, add ice cubes and blend again until well combined.

Pour the antioxidant-rich smoothie into a glass.

Optional: Garnish with a cherry or a sprinkle of chia.

NUTRITIONAL INFORMATION

Calories: 280 kcal, Protein: 12g

Fiber: 8g, Fat: 5g

Carbohydrates: 45g

Peachy Keen Smoothie

INGREDIENTS

1 cup fresh or frozen peach slices

1/2 cup pineapple chunks (fresh or frozen)

1/2 banana

1/2 cup Greek yogurt

1/2 cup coconut water

1 tablespoon flaxseeds

1 teaspoon honey (optional)

Ice cubes (optional)

PREPARATION

In a blender, combine peach slices, pineapple chunks, banana, Greek yogurt, coconut water, and flaxseeds.

Add a teaspoon of honey for a touch of sweetness if preferred.

Blend the mixture on high speed.

For an extra chill, incorporate ice cubes and blend again until well combined.

Pour the refreshing smoothie into a glass.

Optional: Garnish with a peach slice or a drizzle of honey.

NUTRITIONAL INFORMATION

Calories: 270 kcal, Protein: 11g

Fiber: 8g, Fat: 5g

Carbohydrates: 45g

CHAPTER 4: VEGETABLE SMOOTHIES RECIPES

This chapter is a celebration of the diverse flavors that vegetables bring to the table. We delve into the power of greens, roots, and cruciferous wonders to provide you with a variety of options that are both healing and delightful.

Here, we celebrate the vibrant hues and nutritional bounty of nature's finest produce, we embark on a journey through the garden, exploring the earthy flavors and health benefits of vegetables.

From the detoxifying powers of Kale and Pineapple Detox to refreshing Cucumber Spinach.

Enjoy a collection of simple yet satisfying recipes that make it easy to boost your intake of essential nutrients.

So, grab your blender and let's explore the bountiful world of vegetable smoothies together.

Kale and Pineapple Detox Smoothie

INGREDIENTS

1 cup kale leaves, stems removed

1/2 cup pineapple chunks (fresh or frozen)

1/2 banana

1/2 cucumber, peeled and chopped

1/2 cup coconut water

1 tablespoon chia seeds

1 teaspoon ginger, grated

1 teaspoon honey (optional)

Ice cubes (optional)

PREPARATION

In a blender, combine kale leaves, pineapple chunks, banana, cucumber, coconut water, chia seeds, and grated ginger.

If desired, add a teaspoon of honey for a touch of sweetness.

Blend the mixture on high speed.

For an extra chill, include ice cubes and blend again until well combined.

Pour the detoxifying smoothie into a glass.

Optional: Garnish with a slice of cucumber or a sprinkle of chia seeds.

NUTRITIONAL INFORMATION

Calories: 220 kcal, Protein: 7g

Fiber: 8g, Fat: 6g

Carbohydrates: 40g

Carrot-Ginger Smoothie

INGREDIENTS

1/2 cup carrots, peeled and chopped

1/2 banana

1/2 orange, peeled and segmented

1/2 cup Greek yogurt

1/2 cup almond milk

1 teaspoon fresh ginger, grated

1 tablespoon flaxseeds

1 teaspoon honey (optional

Ice cubes (optional)

PREPARATION

In a blender, combine chopped carrots, banana, orange segments, Greek yogurt, almond milk, grated ginger, and flaxseeds.

If desired, add a teaspoon of honey for a touch of sweetness.

Blend the mixture on high speed.

For a cooler consistency, add ice cubes and blend again until well combined.

Pour the revitalizing smoothie into a glass.

Optional: Garnish with a slice of orange or a sprinkle of flaxseeds.

NUTRITIONAL INFORMATION

Calories: 240 kcal, Protein: 10g

Fiber: 7g, Fat: 6g

Carbohydrates: 40g

Green Goddess Glow Smoothie

INGREDIENTS

1 cup spinach leaves, washed

1/2 avocado, peeled and pitted

1/2 banana

1/2 green apple, cored and chopped

1/2 cup cucumber, peeled and chopped

1/2 cup coconut water

1 tablespoon chia seeds

1 teaspoon spirulina powder

1 teaspoon honey (optional)

Ice cubes (optional)

PREPARATION

In a blender, combine spinach leaves, avocado, banana, green apple, cucumber, coconut water, chia seeds, spirulina powder, and honey.

If desired, add a teaspoon of honey for a touch of sweetness.

Blend the mixture on high speed.

For a cooler consistency, add ice cubes and blend again until well combined.

Pour the glowing smoothie into a glass.

Optional: Garnish with a slice of green apple or a sprinkle of chia seeds.

NUTRITIONAL INFORMATION

Calories: 270 kcal, Protein: 8g

Fiber: 9g, Fat: 13g

Carbohydrates: 40g

Carrot Kale Smoothie

INGREDIENTS

1/2 cup carrots, peeled and chopped

1 cup kale leaves, stems removed

1/2 banana

1/2 cup pineapple chunks (fresh or frozen)

1/2 cup Greek yogurt

1/2 cup coconut water

1 tablespoon flaxseeds

1 teaspoon honey (optional)

Ice cubes (optional)

PREPARATION

In a blender, combine chopped carrots, kale leaves, banana, pineapple chunks, Greek yogurt, coconut water, flaxseeds, and honey.

If desired, add a teaspoon of honey for a touch of sweetness.

Blend the mixture on high speed.

For a cooler consistency, add ice cubes and blend again until well combined.

Pour the radiance-boosting smoothie into a glass.

Optional: Garnish with a kale leaf or a slice of pineapple.

NUTRITIONAL INFORMATION

Calories: 240 kcal, Protein: 10g

Fiber: 7g, Fat: 6g

Carbohydrates: 40g

Beetroot Bliss Smoothie

INGREDIENTS

Ingredients:

1/2 cup beets, cooked and chopped

1/2 cup strawberries, hulled (fresh or frozen)

1/2 banana

1/2 cup Greek yogurt

1/2 cup almond milk

1 tablespoon chia seeds

1 teaspoon honey (optional)

Ice cubes (optional)

PREPARATION

In a blender, combine cooked and chopped beets, strawberries, banana, Greek yogurt, almond milk, chia seeds, and honey.

If desired, add a teaspoon of honey for a touch of sweetness.

Blend the mixture on high speed.

For a cooler consistency, add ice cubes and blend again until well combined.

Pour the smoothie into a glass.

Optional: Garnish with a strawberry slice or a drizzle of honey.

NUTRITIONAL INFORMATION

Calories: 250 kcal, Protein: 12g

Fiber: 8g, Fat: 6g

Carbohydrates: 40g

Cucumber Spinach Smoothie

INGREDIENTS

1/2 cucumber, peeled and chopped

1 cup spinach leaves, washed

1/2 banana

1/2 green apple, cored and chopped

1/2 cup Greek yogurt

1/2 cup coconut water

1 tablespoon chia seeds

1 teaspoon honey (optional)

Ice cubes (optional)

PREPARATION

In a blender, combine chopped cucumber, spinach leaves, banana, green apple, Greek yogurt, coconut water, chia seeds, and honey.

If desired, add a teaspoon of honey for a touch of sweetness.

Blend the mixture on high speed.

For an extra chill, include ice cubes and blend again until well combined.

Pour into a glass.

Optional: Garnish with a slice of cucumber or a sprinkle of chia seeds.

NUTRITIONAL INFORMATION

Calories: 230 kcal, Protein: 9g

Fiber: 8g, Fat: 6g

Carbohydrates: 40g

Sweet Pea Zen Zest Smoothie

INGREDIENTS

1/2 cup sweet peas, blanched

1/2 cup pineapple chunks (fresh or frozen)

1/2 banana

1/2 cup spinach leaves, washed

1/2 cup coconut water

1 tablespoon fresh ginger, peeled and grated

1 tablespoon flaxseeds

1 teaspoon honey (optional)

Ice cubes (optional)

PREPARATION

Blanch the sweet peas in boiling water for a minute, then immediately transfer them to an ice bath to cool.

In a blender, combine blanched sweet peas, pineapple chunks, banana, spinach leaves, coconut water, grated ginger, flaxseeds, and honey.

If desired, add a teaspoon of honey for a touch of sweetness.

Blend the mixture on high speed.

For a cooler consistency, add ice cubes and blend again until well combined.

Pour into a glass.

NUTRITIONAL INFORMATION

Calories: 200 kcal, Protein: 6g

Fiber: 8g, Fat: 5g

Carbohydrates: 35g

Asparagus Avocado Smoothie

INGREDIENTS

1/2 cup asparagus, trimmed and steamed

1/2 avocado, peeled and pitted

1/2 banana

1/2 cup pineapple chunks (fresh or frozen)

1/2 cup Greek yogurt

1/2 cup almond milk

1 tablespoon pumpkin seeds

1 teaspoon honey (optional

Ice cubes (optional)

PREPARATION

Trim and steam the asparagus until it's tender, then allow it to cool. In a blender, combine steamed asparagus, avocado, banana, pineapple chunks, Greek yogurt, almond milk, pumpkin seeds, and honey.

If desired, add a teaspoon of honey for a touch of sweetness. Blend the mixture on high speed.

For a cooler consistency, add ice cubes and blend again until well combined. Pour into a glass.

Optional: Garnish with a sprinkle of pumpkin seeds or a slice of pineapple.

NUTRITIONAL INFORMATION

Calories: 280 kcal, Protein: 11g

Fiber: 8g, Fat: 14g

Carbohydrates: 35g

Radish Radiance Smoothie

INGREDIENTS

1 cup radishes, washed and trimmed

1/2 cucumber, peeled and chopped

1/2 green apple, cored and chopped

1/2 lemon, juiced

1/2 cup coconut water

1 tablespoon mint leaves

1 teaspoon chia seeds

1 teaspoon honey (optional

Ice cubes (optional)

PREPARATION

In a blender, combine washed and trimmed radishes, chopped cucumber, green apple, lemon juice, coconut water, mint leaves, chia seeds, and honey.

If desired, add a teaspoon of honey for a touch of sweetness.

Blend the mixture on high speed.

For a cooler consistency, add ice cubes and blend again until well combined.

Pour into a glass.

Optional: Garnish with a mint sprig or a slice of cucumber.

NUTRITIONAL INFORMATION

Calories: 160 kcal, Protein: 3g

Fiber: 6g, Fat: 2g

Carbohydrates: 35g

Butternut Squash Spice Infusion Smoothie

INGREDIENTS

1/2 cup butternut squash, cooked and cubed

1/2 banana

1/2 pear, cored and chopped

1/2 cup Greek yogurt

1/2 cup almond milk

1/2 teaspoon ground cinnamon

1/4 teaspoon ground nutmeg

1 tablespoon flaxseeds

1 teaspoon honey (optional)

Ice cubes (optional)

PREPARATION

Cook butternut squash until it's tender, allow to cool before cubing.

In a blender, combine cooked and cubed butternut squash, banana, pear, Greek yogurt, almond milk, ground cinnamon, ground nutmeg, flaxseeds, and honey. If desired, add a teaspoon of honey. Blend the mixture on high speed.

For a cooler consistency, add ice cubes and blend again. Pour into a glass.

Optional: Garnish with a sprinkle of cinnamon or a slice of pear.

NUTRITIONAL INFORMATION

Calories: 270 kcal, Protein: 10g

Fiber: 9g, Fat: 7g

Carbohydrates: 45g

Broccoli Basil Smoothie

INGREDIENTS

1/2 cup broccoli florets, steamed

1/2 cup pineapple chunks (fresh or frozen)

1/2 banana

1/2 cup fresh basil leaves

1/2 cup Greek yogurt

1/2 cup almond milk

1 tablespoon chia seeds

1 teaspoon honey (optional)

Ice cubes (optional)

PREPARATION

Steam the broccoli florets until they are tender, then allow them to cool.

In a blender, combine steamed broccoli, pineapple chunks, banana, fresh basil leaves, Greek yogurt, almond milk, chia seeds, and honey.

If desired, add a teaspoon of honey for a touch of sweetness. Blend the mixture on high speed. For a cooler consistency, add ice cubes and blend again until well combined.

Pour into a glass.

Optional: Garnish with a basil leaf or a slice of pineapple.

NUTRITIONAL INFORMATION

Calories: 240 kcal, Protein: 11g

Fiber: 7g, Fat: 6g

Carbohydrates: 40g

Spinach Avocado Smoothie

INGREDIENTS

1 cup spinach leaves, washed

1/2 avocado, peeled and pitted

1/2 banana

1/2 cup pineapple chunks (fresh or frozen)

1/2 cup Greek yogurt

1/2 cup almond milk

1 tablespoon chia seeds

1 teaspoon honey (optional)

Ice cubes (optional)

PREPARATION

In a blender, combine spinach leaves, avocado, banana, pineapple chunks, Greek yogurt, almond milk, chia seeds, and honey.

If desired, add a teaspoon of honey for a touch of sweetness.

Blend the mixture on high speed.

For a cooler consistency, add ice cubes and blend again until well combined.

Pour into a glass.

Optional: Garnish with a slice of avocado or a sprinkle of chia seeds.

NUTRITIONAL INFORMATION

Calories: 280 kcal, Protein: 12g

Fiber: 9g, Fat: 14g

Carbohydrates: 40g

Kale Mango Smoothie

INGREDIENTS

1 cup kale leaves, washed and stems removed

1/2 cup mango chunks (fresh or frozen)

1/2 banana

1/2 cup Greek yogurt

1/2 cup coconut water

1 tablespoon hemp seeds

1 teaspoon honey (optional)

Ice cubes (optional)

PREPARATION

In a blender, combine kale leaves, mango chunks, banana, Greek yogurt, coconut water, hemp seeds, and honey.

If desired, add a teaspoon of honey for a touch of sweetness.

Blend the mixture on high speed.

For a cooler consistency, add ice cubes and blend again until well combined.

Pour the smoothie into a glass.

Optional: Garnish with a mango slice or a sprinkle of hemp seeds.

NUTRITIONAL INFORMATION

Calories: 260 kcal, Protein: 10g

Fiber: 8g, Fat: 6g

Carbohydrates: 40g

Celery Cilantro Smoothie

INGREDIENTS

2 celery stalks, washed and chopped

1/2 cup fresh cilantro leaves, washed

1/2 cucumber, peeled and chopped

1/2 green apple, cored and chopped

1/2 lemon, juiced

1/2 cup coconut water

1 tablespoon chia seeds

1 teaspoon honey (optional

Ice cubes (optional)

PREPARATION

In a blender, combine chopped celery, cilantro leaves, cucumber, green apple, lemon juice, coconut water, chia seeds, and honey.

If desired, add a teaspoon of honey for a touch of sweetness.

Blend the mixture on high speed.

For a cooler consistency, add ice cubes and blend again until well combined.

Pour into a glass.

Optional: Garnish with a cilantro sprig or a slice of cucumber.

NUTRITIONAL INFORMATION

Calories: 180 kcal, Protein: 4g

Fiber: 7g, Fat: 5g

Carbohydrates: 35g

CHAPTER 5: PROTEIN-PACKED SMOOTHIES RECIPES

Maintaining strength and energy levels is crucial, especially during cancer treatment. That is why we have crafted a collection of recipes that provides the protein punch your body needs. These elixirs are more than just beverages; they are a source of sustenance and vitality.

Proteins are the building blocks of life, and incorporating them into your diet is essential for repairing and regenerating tissues. Whether you opt for the Greek Yogurt Berry, the Plant-Based Protein Paradise, or the Peanut Butter Banana, you are not just enjoying a smoothie; you are embracing a nutritional powerhouse that supports your well-being.

Almond Butter Banana Boost Smoothie

INGREDIENTS

1 banana

1 tablespoon almond butter

1/2 cup Greek yogurt

1/2 cup almond milk

1 tablespoon hemp seeds

1 teaspoon honey (optional)

Ice cubes (optional)

PREPARATION

Peel and slice the banana.

In a blender, combine banana slices, almond butter, Greek yogurt, almond milk, hemp seeds, and honey.

If desired, add a teaspoon of honey.

Blend the mixture on high speed.

For a cooler consistency, add ice cubes and blend again until well combined.

Pour into a glass.

Optional: Garnish with a sprinkle of hemp seeds or a drizzle of almond butter.

NUTRITIONAL INFORMATION

Calories: 300 kcal, Protein: 12g

Fiber: 5g, Fat: 15g

Carbohydrates: 35g

Greek Yogurt Berry Smoothie

INGREDIENTS

1/2 cup mixed berries (strawberries, blueberries, raspberries)

1/2 cup Greek yogurt

1/2 banana

1/2 cup almond milk

1 tablespoon chia seeds

1 teaspoon honey (optional)

Ice cubes (optional)

PREPARATION

Wash the mixed berries thoroughly. In a blender, combine mixed berries, Greek yogurt, banana, almond milk, chia seeds, and honey.

If desired, add a teaspoon of honey.

Blend the mixture on high speed.

For a cooler consistency, add ice cubes and blend again until well combined.

Pour into a glass.

Optional: Garnish with a few whole berries or a sprinkle of chia seeds.

NUTRITIONAL INFORMATION

Calories: 220 kcal, Protein: 10g

Fiber: 6g, Fat: 8g

Carbohydrates: 30g

Plant-Based Protein Paradise Smoothie

INGREDIENTS

1/2 cup silken tofu

1/2 cup edamame, shelled

1/2 banana

1/2 cup spinach leaves, washed

1/2 cup almond milk

1 tablespoon almond butter

1 tablespoon chia seeds

1 teaspoon maple syrup (optional)

Ice cubes (optional)

PREPARATION

In a blender, combine silken tofu, shelled edamame, banana, spinach leaves, almond milk, almond butter, chia seeds, and maple syrup.

If preferred, add a teaspoon of maple syrup.

Blend the mixture on high speed.

For a cooler consistency, add ice cubes and blend again until well combined.

Pour into a glass.

Optional: Garnish with a sprinkle of chia seeds or a drizzle of almond butter.

NUTRITIONAL INFORMATION

Calories: 300 kcal, Protein: 18g

Fiber: 8g, Fat: 14g

Carbohydrates: 30g

Protein Power Berry Smoothie

INGREDIENTS

1/2 cup mixed berries (strawberries, blueberries, raspberries)

1/2 cup Greek yogurt

1/2 cup cottage cheese

1/2 banana

1/2 cup almond milk

1 tablespoon hemp seeds

1 teaspoon honey (optional)

Ice cubes (optional)

PREPARATION

Wash the mixed berries thoroughly. In a blender, combine mixed berries, Greek yogurt, cottage cheese, banana, almond milk, hemp seeds, and honey.

If desired, add a teaspoon of honey.

Blend the mixture on high speed.

For a cooler consistency, add ice cubes and blend again until well combined.

Pour into a glass.

Optional: Garnish with a few whole berries or a sprinkle of hemp seeds.

NUTRITIONAL INFORMATION

Calories: 280 kcal, Protein: 20g

Fiber: 6g, Fat: 12g

Carbohydrates: 25g

Peanut Butter Banana Smoothie

INGREDIENTS

1 banana

2 tablespoons peanut butter (unsweetened)

1/2 cup Greek yogurt

1/2 cup almond milk

1 tablespoon flaxseeds

1 teaspoon honey (optional)

Ice cubes (optional)

PREPARATION

Peel and slice the banana.

In a blender, combine banana slices, peanut butter, Greek yogurt, almond milk, flaxseeds, and honey.

If desired, add a teaspoon of honey.

Blend the mixture on high speed.

For a cooler consistency, add ice cubes and blend again until well combined.

Pour into a glass.

Optional: Garnish with a sprinkle of flaxseeds or a drizzle of peanut butter.

NUTRITIONAL INFORMATION

Calories: 350 kcal, Protein: 12g

Fiber: 6g, Fat: 20g

Carbohydrates: 35g

Chia Seed Chocolate Smoothie

INGREDIENTS

1 cup almond milk (unsweetened)

2 tablespoons chia seeds

1 tablespoon cocoa powder (unsweetened)

1/2 banana

1 tablespoon almond butter

1 teaspoon honey (optional)

Ice cubes (optional)

PREPARATION

In a blender, combine almond milk and chia seeds. Allow the chia seeds to soak in almond milk for at least 15 minutes to create a chia gel.

Peel and slice the banana. Add cocoa powder, banana slices, almond butter, and honey to the blender. If desired, add a teaspoon of honey. Blend the mixture on high speed.

For a cooler consistency, add ice cubes and blend again until well combined. Pour into a glass.

Optional: Garnish with a drizzle of almond butter or a sprinkle of cocoa powder.

NUTRITIONAL INFORMATION

Calories: 300 kcal, Protein: 8g

Fiber: 14g, Fat: 16g

Carbohydrates: 35g

Cashew Coconut Creamy Smoothie

INGREDIENTS

1/2 cup cashews (soaked overnight or at least soaked for 4 hours)

1/2 cup coconut milk (unsweetened)

1/2 banana

1/4 cup shredded coconut (unsweetened)

1 tablespoon chia seeds

1 teaspoon agave syrup (optional)

Ice cubes (optional)

PREPARATION

Drain the soaked cashews and rinse them thoroughly.

In a blender, combine soaked cashews, coconut milk, banana, shredded coconut, chia seeds, and agave syrup.

If desired, add a teaspoon of agave syrup. Blend the mixture on high speed.

For a cooler consistency, add ice cubes and blend again until well combined.

Pour into a glass.

Optional: Garnish with a sprinkle of shredded coconut or a few crushed cashews.

NUTRITIONAL INFORMATION

Calories: 400 kcal, Protein: 8g

Fiber: 6g, Fat: 30g

Carbohydrates: 25g

Quinoa Blueberry Smoothie

INGREDIENTS

1/4 cup cooked quinoa (cooled)

1/2 cup blueberries (fresh or frozen)

1/2 banana

1/2 cup Greek yogurt

1/2 cup almond milk

1 tablespoon flaxseeds

1 teaspoon honey (optional)

Ice cubes (optional)

PREPARATION

Allow the quinoa to cool after cooking according to package instructions. In a blender, combine cooked quinoa, blueberries, banana, Greek yogurt, almond milk, flaxseeds, and honey.

If desired, add a teaspoon of honey.

Blend the mixture on high speed.

For a cooler consistency, add ice cubes and blend again until well combined.

Pour into a glass.

Optional: Garnish with a few whole blueberries or a sprinkle

NUTRITIONAL INFORMATION

Calories: 300 kcal, Protein: 12g

Fiber: 8g, Fat: 8g

Carbohydrates: 45g

Hemp Heart Healer Smoothie

INGREDIENTS

1 tablespoon hemp hearts

1/2 cup strawberries (fresh or frozen)

1/2 banana

1/2 cup kale leaves, stems removed

1/2 cup almond milk

1 tablespoon almond butter

1 teaspoon maple syrup (optional)

Ice cubes (optional)

PREPARATION

In a blender, combine hemp hearts, strawberries, banana, kale leaves, almond milk, almond butter, and maple syrup.

If preferred, add a teaspoon of maple syrup.

Blend the mixture on high speed.

For a cooler consistency, add ice cubes and blend again until well combined.

Pour into a glass.

Optional: Garnish with a few sliced strawberries or a sprinkle of hemp hearts.

NUTRITIONAL INFORMATION

Calories: 250 kcal, Protein: 8g

Fiber: 6g, Fat: 12g

Carbohydrates: 30g

Pumpkin Seed Protein Smoothie

INGREDIENTS

2 tablespoons pumpkin seeds (pepitas)

1/2 cup pineapple chunks (fresh or frozen)

1/2 banana

1/2 cup spinach leaves, washed

1/2 cup coconut water

1 tablespoon coconut oil

1 teaspoon agave syrup (optional)

Ice cubes (optional)

PREPARATION

In a blender, combine pumpkin seeds, pineapple chunks, banana, spinach leaves, coconut water, coconut oil, and agave syrup.

If desired, add a teaspoon of agave syrup.

Blend the mixture on high speed.

For a cooler consistency, add ice cubes and blend again until well combined.

Pour into a glass.

Optional: Garnish with a few pumpkin seeds or a slice of pineapple.

NUTRITIONAL INFORMATION

Calories: 300 kcal, Protein: 10g

Fiber: 6g, Fat: 15g

Carbohydrates: 35g

Flaxseed Fusion Smoothie

INGREDIENTS

1 tablespoon ground flaxseeds

1/2 cup mango chunks (fresh or frozen)

1/2 cup strawberries (fresh or frozen)

1/2 cup cucumber, peeled and chopped

1/2 cup plain yogurt

1 tablespoon honey

1/2 lime, juiced

Ice cubes (optional)

PREPARATION

In a blender, combine ground flaxseeds, mango chunks, strawberries, cucumber, plain yogurt, honey, and lime juice.

Blend the mixture on high speed.

For a cooler consistency, add ice cubes and blend again until well combined.

Pour into a glass.

Optional: Garnish with a slice of lime or a few sliced strawberries.

NUTRITIONAL INFORMATION

Calories: 250 kcal, Protein: 6g

Fiber: 8g, Fat: 7g

Carbohydrates: 45g

Tofu Berry Smoothie

INGREDIENTS

1/2 cup firm tofu, cubed

1/2 cup mixed berries (blueberries, raspberries, strawberries)

1/2 banana

1/2 cup almond milk

1 tablespoon almond butter

1 teaspoon agave syrup (optional)

Ice cubes (optional)

PREPARATION

In a blender, combine cubed firm tofu, mixed berries, banana, almond milk, almond butter, and agave syrup.

If desired, add a teaspoon of agave syrup.

Blend the mixture on high speed.

For a cooler consistency, add ice cubes and blend again until well combined.

Pour into a glass.

Optional: Garnish with a few whole berries or a drizzle of almond butter.

NUTRITIONAL INFORMATION

Calories: 300 kcal, Protein: 14g

Fiber: 8g, Fat: 15g

Carbohydrates: 35g

Chickpea Cinnamon Smoothie

INGREDIENTS

1/2 cup cooked chickpeas (canned or boiled)

1/2 cup apple slices

1/2 banana

1/2 cup unsweetened almond milk

1/2 teaspoon ground cinnamon

1 tablespoon honey

Ice cubes (optional)

PREPARATION

In a blender, combine cooked chickpeas, apple slices, banana, almond milk, ground cinnamon, and honey.

Blend the mixture on high speed.

For a cooler consistency, add ice cubes and blend again until well combined.

Pour into a glass.

Optional: Garnish with a sprinkle of ground cinnamon or a few apple slices.

NUTRITIONAL INFORMATION

Calories: 300 kcal, Protein: 10g

Fiber: 8g, Fat: 5g

Carbohydrates: 55g

Lentil Lime Lusciousness Smoothie

INGREDIENTS

1/4 cup cooked lentils (canned or boiled)

1/2 cup pineapple chunks (fresh or frozen)

1/2 banana

1/2 lime, juiced

1/2 cup coconut water

1 tablespoon coconut flakes

1 teaspoon maple syrup (optional)

Ice cubes (optional)

PREPARATION

In a blender, combine cooked lentils, pineapple chunks, banana, lime juice, coconut water, coconut flakes, and optional maple syrup.

Blend the mixture on high speed.

For a cooler consistency, add ice cubes and blend again until well combined.

Pour into a glass.

Optional: Garnish with a slice of lime or a sprinkle of coconut flakes.

NUTRITIONAL INFORMATION

Calories: 250 kcal, Protein: 9g

Fiber: 8g, Fat: 5g

Carbohydrates: 45g

CHAPTER 6: HYDRATION AND HEALING SMOOTHIES RECIPES

Join us on this liquid journey, where we have blended the art of hydration with the science of nutrition. We understand that the journey through breast cancer treatment may present challenges, and adequate hydration becomes paramount.

Staying adequately hydrated is fundamental to your well-being, and we have curated a collection of smoothie recipes that not only quench your thirst but also provide a therapeutic boost during your journey to recovery.

Hydration is the cornerstone of vitality, and our smoothie creations are designed to be more than just delicious beverages.

In this chapter, we explore the revitalizing properties of ingredients like watermelon, cucumber, and mint, crafting smoothies that serve as a healing elixir for your body and soul.

Coconut Water Refresh Smoothie

INGREDIENTS

1/2 cup coconut water

1/2 cup cucumber, peeled and chopped

1/2 cup pineapple chunks (fresh or frozen)

1/2 cup green grapes

1/2 lime, juiced

1 tablespoon fresh mint leaves

1 teaspoon honey

Ice cubes (optional)

PREPARATION

In a blender, combine coconut water, chopped cucumber, pineapple chunks, green grapes, lime juice, fresh mint leaves, and honey.

Blend the mixture on high speed.

For a cooler consistency, add ice cubes and blend again until well combined.

Pour the smoothie into a glass.

Optional: Garnish with a sprig of mint or a slice of lime.

NUTRITIONAL INFORMATION

Calories: 150 kcal, Protein: 2g

Fiber: 3g, Fat: 0g

Carbohydrates: 40g

Cucumber Mint Smoothie

INGREDIENTS

1/2 cup cucumber, peeled and chopped

1/2 cup honeydew melon, diced

1/2 cup green grapes

1/2 lime, juiced

1/2 cup coconut water

1 tablespoon fresh mint leaves

1 teaspoon agave syrup (optional)

Ice cubes (optional)

PREPARATION

In a blender, combine chopped cucumber, diced honeydew melon, green grapes, lime juice, coconut water, fresh mint leaves, and optional agave syrup.

Blend the mixture on high speed.

For a cooler consistency, add ice cubes and blend again until well combined.

Pour into a glass.

Optional: Garnish with a sprig of mint or a slice of cucumber.

NUTRITIONAL INFORMATION

Calories: 120 kcal, Protein: 2g

Fiber: 3g, Fat: 0g

Carbohydrates: 30g

Green Tea Infusion Smoothie

INGREDIENTS

1/2 cup green tea, brewed and cooled

1/2 cup pineapple chunks (fresh or frozen)

1/2 cup spinach leaves

1/2 banana

1/2 teaspoon matcha powder

1 tablespoon chia seeds

1 teaspoon honey (optional)

Ice cubes (optional)

PREPARATION

Brew green tea and allow it cool down to room temperature.

In a blender, combine cooled green tea, pineapple chunks, spinach leaves, banana, matcha powder, chia seeds, and optional honey.

Blend the mixture on high speed.

For a cooler consistency, add ice cubes and blend again until well combined.

Pour into a glass.

Optional: Garnish with a sprinkle of matcha powder or a slice of pineapple.

NUTRITIONAL INFORMATION

Calories: 150 kcal, Protein: 3g

Fiber: 5g, Fat: 3g

Carbohydrates: 30g

Watermelon Mint Smoothie

INGREDIENTS

1 cup watermelon, diced (seedless)

1/2 cup cucumber, peeled and chopped

1/2 lime, juiced

1 tablespoon fresh mint leaves

1/2 cup coconut water

1 teaspoon agave syrup (optional)

Ice cubes (optional)

PREPARATION

In a blender, combine diced watermelon, chopped cucumber, lime juice, fresh mint leaves, coconut water, and optional agave syrup.

Blend the mixture on high speed.

For a cooler consistency, add ice cubes and blend again until well combined.

Pour into a glass.

Optional: Garnish with a sprig of mint or a slice of watermelon.

NUTRITIONAL INFORMATION

Calories: 100 kcal, Protein: 1g

Fiber: 2g, Fat: 0g

Carbohydrates: 25g

Celery Hydration Smoothie

INGREDIENTS

1/2 cup celery, chopped

1/2 cup cucumber, peeled and chopped

1/2 green apple, cored and chopped

1/2 lemon, juiced

1/2 cup coconut water

1 tablespoon fresh parsley leaves

1 teaspoon honey (optional)

Ice cubes (optional)

PREPARATION

In a blender, combine chopped celery, chopped cucumber, chopped green apple, lemon juice, coconut water, fresh parsley leaves, and optional honey.

Blend the mixture on high speed.

For a cooler consistency, add ice cubes and blend again until well combined.

Pour into a glass.

Optional: Garnish with a sprig of parsley or a slice of lemon.

NUTRITIONAL INFORMATION

Calories: 80 kcal, Protein: 1g

Fiber: 3g, Fat: 0g

Carbohydrates: 20g

Blueberry Coconut Smoothie

INGREDIENTS

1/2 cup blueberries (fresh or frozen)

1/2 banana

1/2 cup Greek yogurt

1/2 cup coconut water

1 tablespoon shredded coconut

1 teaspoon chia seeds

1 teaspoon honey (optional)

Ice cubes (optional)

PREPARATION

In a blender, combine blueberries, banana, Greek yogurt, coconut water, shredded coconut, chia seeds, and optional honey.

Blend the mixture on high speed.

For a cooler consistency, add ice cubes and blend again until well combined.

Pour into a glass.

Optional: Garnish with a sprinkle of shredded coconut or a few fresh blueberries.

NUTRITIONAL INFORMATION

Calories: 200 kcal, Protein: 6g

Fiber: 5g, Fat: 8g

Carbohydrates: 30g

Citrus Hydrating Burst Smoothie

INGREDIENTS

1/2 cup orange segments

1/2 cup grapefruit segments

1/2 cup pineapple chunks

1/2 cup cucumber, peeled and chopped

1/2 lime, juiced

1/2 cup coconut water

1 teaspoon honey (optional)

Ice cubes (optional)

PREPARATION

In a blender, combine orange segments, grapefruit segments, pineapple chunks, chopped cucumber, lime juice, coconut water, and optional honey.

Blend the mixture on high.

For a cooler consistency, add ice cubes and blend again until well combined.

Pour into a glass.

Optional: Garnish with a slice of orange or a wedge of lime.

NUTRITIONAL INFORMATION

Calories: 120 kcal, Protein: 2g

Fiber: 3g, Fat: 0g

Carbohydrates: 30g

Pineapple Basil Infusion Smoothie

INGREDIENTS

1/2 cup pineapple chunks

1/2 banana

1/2 cup Greek yogurt

1/2 cup coconut water

1/4 cup fresh basil leaves

1 tablespoon flaxseeds

1 teaspoon honey (optional)

Ice cubes (optional)

PREPARATION

In a blender, combine pineapple chunks, banana, Greek yogurt, coconut water, fresh basil leaves, flaxseeds, and optional honey.

Blend the mixture on high speed.

For a cooler consistency, add ice cubes and blend again until well combined.

Pour into a glass.

Optional: Garnish with a sprig of basil or a few pineapple chunks.

NUTRITIONAL INFORMATION

Calories: 180 kcal, Protein: 6g

Fiber: 4g, Fat: 6g

Carbohydrates: 28g

Cranberry Hydration Smoothie

INGREDIENTS

1/2 cup cranberries (fresh or unsweetened frozen)

1/2 cup cucumber, peeled and chopped

1/2 cup watermelon, diced

1/2 cup coconut water

1 tablespoon chia seeds

1 teaspoon fresh mint leaves

1 teaspoon honey (optional)

Ice cubes (optional)

PREPARATION

In a blender, combine cranberries, chopped cucumber, diced watermelon, coconut water, chia seeds, fresh mint leaves, and optional honey.

Blend the mixture on high speed.

For a cooler consistency, add ice cubes and blend again until well combined.

Pour into a glass.

Optional: Garnish with a sprig of mint or a few cranberries.

NUTRITIONAL INFORMATION

Calories: 100 kcal, Protein: 2g

Fiber: 5g, Fat: 3g

Carbohydrates: 20g

Lemon Ginger Healing Splash Smoothie

INGREDIENTS

1/2 lemon, peeled and segmented

1/2 inch fresh ginger, peeled and grated

1/2 cup pineapple chunks

1/2 banana

1/2 cup Greek yogurt

1/2 cup coconut water

1 teaspoon honey (optional)

Ice cubes (optional)

PREPARATION

In a blender, combine lemon segments, grated ginger, pineapple chunks, banana, Greek yogurt, coconut water, and optional honey.

Blend the mixture on high speed.

For a cooler consistency, add ice cubes and blend again until well combined.

Pour into a glass.

Optional: Garnish with a slice of lemon or a sprinkle of grated ginger.

NUTRITIONAL INFORMATION

Calories: 150 kcal, Protein: 6g

Fiber: 3g, Fat: 3g

Carbohydrates: 30g

Melon Mint Smoothie

INGREDIENTS

1/2 cup honeydew melon, diced

1/2 cup cantaloupe, diced

1/2 cup cucumber, peeled and chopped

1/4 cup fresh mint leaves

1/2 lime, juiced

1/2 cup coconut water

1 teaspoon honey (optional)

Ice cubes (optional)

PREPARATION

In a blender, combine honeydew melon, cantaloupe, chopped cucumber, fresh mint leaves, lime juice, coconut water, and optional honey.

Blend the mixture on high speed.

For a cooler consistency, add ice cubes and blend again until well combined.

Pour into a glass.

Optional: Garnish with a sprig of mint or a few melon balls.

NUTRITIONAL INFORMATION

Calories: 90 kcal, Protein: 2g

Fiber: 3g, Fat: 0g

Carbohydrates: 22g

Green Grape Smoothie

INGREDIENTS

1 cup green grapes, stems removed

1/2 green apple, cored and chopped

1/2 cup cucumber, peeled and sliced

1/2 cup spinach leaves

1/2 lemon, juiced

1/2 cup coconut water

1 teaspoon chia seeds

Ice cubes (optional)

PREPARATION

In a blender, combine green grapes, chopped green apple, sliced cucumber, spinach leaves, lemon juice, coconut water, and chia seeds.

Blend the mixture on high speed.

For a cooler consistency, add ice cubes and blend again until well combined.

Pour into a glass.

Optional: Garnish with a slice of green apple or a few whole grapes.

NUTRITIONAL INFORMATION

Calories: 120 kcal, Protein: 2g

Fiber: 5g, Fat: 1g

Carbohydrates: 30g

Kiwi Coconut Smoothie

INGREDIENTS

2 kiwis, peeled and sliced

1/2 banana

1/2 cup coconut water

1/4 cup Greek yogurt

1 tablespoon chia seeds

1 teaspoon honey (optional)

Ice cubes (optional)

PREPARATION

In a blender, combine sliced kiwis, banana, coconut water, Greek yogurt, chia seeds, and optional honey.

Blend the mixture on high speed.

For a cooler consistency, add ice cubes and blend again until well combined.

Pour into a glass.

Optional: Garnish with a slice of kiwi or a sprinkle of chia seeds.

NUTRITIONAL INFORMATION

Calories: 160 kcal, Protein: 4g

Fiber: 6g, Fat: 3g

Carbohydrates: 32g

Pomegranate Hydration Harmony Smoothie

INGREDIENTS

1/2 cup pomegranate seeds

1/2 cup cucumber, peeled and sliced

1/2 cup watermelon, diced

1/4 cup fresh mint leaves

1/2 lime, juiced

1/2 cup coconut water

1 teaspoon agave nectar or honey (optional)

Ice cubes (optional)

PREPARATION

In a blender, combine pomegranate seeds, sliced cucumber, diced watermelon, fresh mint leaves, lime juice, coconut water, and optional agave nectar or honey.

Blend the mixture on high speed.

For a cooler consistency, add ice cubes and blend again until well combined.

Pour the smoothie into a glass.

Optional: Garnish with a sprig of mint or a few pomegranate seeds.

NUTRITIONAL INFORMATION

Calories: 90 kcal, Protein: 2g

Fiber: 4g, Fat: 0g

Carbohydrates: 22g

CHAPTER 7: CALMING AND SOOTHING SMOOTHIES RECIPES

This chapter is dedicated to providing you with a moment of tranquility through the art of blending.

From the Lavender Blueberry to the Chamomile Peach, each recipe is a harmonious blend of flavors designed to bring you comfort and peace.

The ingredients chosen for this chapter are not only delicious but also renowned for their calming properties. Lavender, chamomile, and mint are incorporated to create a sensory experience that goes beyond taste.

Imagine the soft aroma of lavender mingling with the sweetness of blueberries or the refreshing mint dancing with the subtle notes of melon. So slow down, take a deep breath, and enjoy every flavor.

Lavender Blueberry Smoothie

INGREDIENTS

1/2 cup blueberries, fresh or frozen

1/2 banana

1/2 cup plain Greek yogurt

1/2 teaspoon dried lavender buds (culinary grade)

1 tablespoon flaxseeds

1/2 cup almond milk

1 teaspoon honey or maple syrup (optional)

Ice cubes (optional)

PREPARATION

In a blender, combine blueberries, banana, Greek yogurt, dried lavender buds, flaxseeds, almond milk, and optional honey or maple syrup.

Blend the mixture on high speed.

For a cooler consistency, add ice cubes and blend again until well combined.

Pour into a glass.

Optional: Garnish with a sprinkle of dried lavender buds.

NUTRITIONAL INFORMATION

Calories: 180 kcal, Protein: 8g

Fiber: 5g, Fat: 6g

Carbohydrates: 25g

Chamomile Peach Smoothie

INGREDIENTS

1 ripe peach, pitted and sliced

1/2 cup frozen mango chunks

1/2 cup chamomile tea, brewed and chilled

1/2 cup vanilla Greek yogurt

1 tablespoon chia seeds

1 teaspoon honey (optional)

Ice cubes (optional)

PREPARATION

Brew a cup of chamomile tea and allow to cool down.

In a blender, combine sliced peach, frozen mango chunks, chilled chamomile tea, vanilla Greek yogurt, chia seeds, and optional honey.

Blend the mixture on high speed.

For a cooler consistency, add ice cubes and blend again until well combined.

Pour into a glass.

NUTRITIONAL INFORMATION

Calories: 200 kcal, Protein: 10g

Fiber: 6g, Fat: 4g

Carbohydrates: 35g

Minty Melon Relaxation Smoothie

INGREDIENTS

1 cup honeydew melon, cubed

1/2 cup cucumber, peeled and sliced

1/2 cup fresh spinach leaves

1/4 cup fresh mint leaves

1/2 cup coconut water

1/2 lime, juiced

1 teaspoon chia seeds

Ice cubes (optional)

PREPARATION

In a blender, combine honeydew melon cubes, cucumber slices, fresh spinach leaves, mint leaves, coconut water, lime juice, and chia seeds.

Blend the mixture on high speed.

For a cooler consistency, add ice cubes and blend again until well combined.

Pour into a glass.

NUTRITIONAL INFORMATION

Calories: 120 kcal, Protein: 3g

Fiber: 5g, Fat: 1g

Carbohydrates: 28g

Lavender Lemon Smoothie

INGREDIENTS

1 cup frozen blueberries

1/2 banana, peeled and sliced

1/2 cup Greek yogurt (plain or vanilla)

1/2 cup almond milk

1 tablespoon fresh lemon juice

1 teaspoon dried lavender buds (culinary-grade)

1 teaspoon honey (optional)

Ice cubes (optional)

PREPARATION

In a blender, combine frozen blueberries, sliced banana, Greek yogurt, almond milk, fresh lemon juice, and dried lavender buds.

Blend the mixture on high speed.

For a cooler consistency, add ice cubes and blend again until well combined.

Taste the smoothie and add honey if preferred.

Pour into a glass.

NUTRITIONAL INFORMATION

Calories: 180 kcal, Protein: 8g

Fiber: 5g, Fat: 4g

Carbohydrates: 30g

Ginger Turmeric Smoothie

INGREDIENTS

1 cup mango chunks (fresh or frozen)

1/2 banana, peeled and sliced

1/2 cup pineapple chunks

1/2 teaspoon fresh ginger, grated

1/2 teaspoon ground turmeric

1 cup coconut water

1 tablespoon chia seeds

Ice cubes (optional)

PREPARATION

In a blender, combine mango chunks, sliced banana, pineapple chunks, grated fresh ginger, and ground turmeric.

Pour in coconut water.

Add chia seeds for an extra boost of omega-3 fatty acids and fiber.

If a cooler temperature is preferred, include ice cubes and blend until well combined.

Pour into a glass.

NUTRITIONAL INFORMATION

Calories: 220 kcal, Protein: 4g

Fiber: 8g, Fat: 3g

Carbohydrates: 45g

Vanilla Chai Smoothie

INGREDIENTS

1 cup brewed chai tea, cooled

1/2 cup almond milk

1/2 banana, peeled and sliced

1/2 teaspoon vanilla extract

1 tablespoon flaxseeds

1 tablespoon honey or maple syrup (optional)

Ice cubes (optional)

PREPARATION

Brew a cup of chai tea and allow it to cool to room temperature.

In a blender, combine the cooled chai tea, almond milk, sliced banana, vanilla extract, and flaxseeds.

Add honey or maple syrup if desired.

For a chilled experience, include ice cubes and blend until well combined.

Pour into a glass.

NUTRITIONAL INFORMATION

Calories: 180 kcal, Protein: 3g

Fiber: 6g, Fat: 7g

Carbohydrates: 28g

Cinnamon Coconut Smoothie

INGREDIENTS

1 cup coconut milk

1/2 cup Greek yogurt

1/2 banana, peeled and frozen

1/2 teaspoon ground cinnamon

1 tablespoon chia seeds

1 tablespoon shredded coconut

Honey or maple syrup (optional)

Ice cubes (optional)

PREPARATION

In a blender, combine coconut milk, Greek yogurt, frozen banana, ground cinnamon, chia seeds, and shredded coconut.

Add honey or maple syrup.

Include ice cubes if you prefer a chilled consistency and blend until smooth.

Pour into a glass.

NUTRITIONAL INFORMATION

Calories: 250 kcal, Protein: 8g

Fiber: 7g, Fat: 18g

Carbohydrates: 17g

Peppermint Pineapple Smoothie

INGREDIENTS

1 cup fresh pineapple chunks

1/2 cup cucumber, peeled and diced

1/2 banana, peeled

1/4 cup fresh mint leaves

1/2 teaspoon peppermint extract

1 tablespoon chia seeds

1 cup coconut water

Ice cubes (optional)

PREPARATION

In a blender, combine fresh pineapple chunks, diced cucumber, peeled banana, mint leaves, peppermint extract, and chia seeds.

Pour in coconut water.

Include ice cubes if you prefer a chilled consistency and blend until smooth.

Pour into a glass.

NUTRITIONAL INFORMATION

Calories: 180 kcal, Protein: 3g

Fiber: 8g, Fat: 4g

Carbohydrates: 35g

Rosemary Berry Smoothie

INGREDIENTS

1/2 cup mixed berries (strawberries, blueberries, raspberries)

1/2 banana, peeled

1/4 cup Greek yogurt

1 teaspoon fresh rosemary leaves

1 tablespoon honey (optional)

1/2 cup almond milk

Ice cubes (optional)

PREPARATION

Combine mixed berries, peeled banana, Greek yogurt, fresh rosemary leaves, and honey (if desired) in a blender.

Pour in almond milk and blend all the ingredients until smooth.

If you prefer a colder smoothie, add ice cubes and blend again until well incorporated.

Pour into a glass.

NUTRITIONAL INFORMATION

Calories: 200 kcal, Protein: 6g

Fiber: 5g, Fat: 4g

Carbohydrates: 35g

Cardamom Carrot Smoothie

INGREDIENTS

1 medium-sized carrot, peeled and chopped

1/2 banana, peeled

1/4 cup Greek yogurt

1/2 teaspoon ground cardamom

1 tablespoon honey (optional)

1/2 cup coconut water

Ice cubes (optional)

PREPARATION

Place chopped carrot, peeled banana, Greek yogurt, ground cardamom, and honey (if desired) into a blender.

Add coconut water and blend all the ingredients until well combined.

For a colder texture, include ice cubes and blend again.

Pour into a glass.

NUTRITIONAL INFORMATION

Calories: 180 kcal, Protein: 5g

Fiber: 4g, Fat: 2g

Carbohydrates: 38g

Basil Peach Smoothie

INGREDIENTS

1 ripe peach, pitted and sliced

1/2 cup fresh basil leaves

1/2 cup plain Greek yogurt

1 tablespoon honey (optional)

1/2 cup almond milk

Ice cubes (optional)

PREPARATION

In a blender, combine the sliced ripe peach, fresh basil leaves, Greek yogurt, and honey.

Add almond milk.

If a colder texture is desired, include ice cubes and blend until well incorporated.

Pour into a glass.

NUTRITIONAL INFORMATION

Calories: 220 kcal, Protein: 10g

Fiber: 3g, Fat: 7g

Carbohydrates: 30g

Turmeric Ginger Smoothie

INGREDIENTS

1 banana, peeled and sliced

1/2 teaspoon ground turmeric

1 teaspoon fresh ginger, grated

1 cup coconut water

1/2 cup frozen mango chunks

1 tablespoon chia seeds

Ice cubes (optional)

PREPARATION

In a blender, combine the sliced banana, ground turmeric, grated ginger, coconut water, frozen mango chunks, and chia seeds.

If a colder texture is preferred, add ice cubes to the blender.

Blend the ingredients until smooth and creamy.

Pour into a glass.

NUTRITIONAL INFORMATION

Calories: 220 kcal, Protein: 4g

Fiber: 8g, Fat: 3g

Carbohydrates: 49g

CHAPTER 8: IMMUNE-BOOSTING ELIXIRS SMOOTHIES RECIPES

These vibrant concoctions serve as guardians of your well-being, empowering your body. Your immune system is the silent warrior that tirelessly protects you, and during times of healing, it deserves an extra boost.

Here you will find a repertoire of smoothie recipes designed to fortify your defenses and infuse your body with the goodness it craves with ingredients carefully selected for their immune-boosting properties such as the Spirulina Citrus Fortification, a vibrant green elixir that brings together the antioxidant prowess of spirulina with the zesty kick of citrus.

These recipes are invitations to a symbiotic dance between ingredients and your body's natural resilience leaving you feeling revitalized and strengthened.

Turmeric Golden Milkshake Smoothie

INGREDIENTS

1 cup almond milk

1/2 teaspoon ground turmeric

1/4 teaspoon ground cinnamon

1/8 teaspoon ground ginger

1/2 frozen banana

1 tablespoon chia seeds

1 teaspoon honey or maple syrup (optional)

Ice cubes (optional)

PREPARATION

In a blender, combine almond milk, ground turmeric, ground cinnamon, ground ginger, frozen banana, chia seeds, and honey or maple syrup if desired.

If you prefer a colder consistency, add ice cubes to the blender.

Blend the ingredients until smooth and creamy.

Pour into a glass.

NUTRITIONAL INFORMATION

Calories: 180 kcal, Protein: 4g

Fiber: 7g, Fat: 7g

Carbohydrates: 26g

Matcha Immuni-Tea Blend Smoothie

INGREDIENTS

1 cup green tea, brewed and cooled

1/2 teaspoon matcha powder

1/2 cup frozen mango chunks

1/2 cup spinach leaves

1/4 avocado

1 tablespoon chia seeds

1 teaspoon honey or agave syrup (optional)

Ice cubes (optional)

PREPARATION

Brew a cup of green tea and allow it cool down to room temperature.

In a blender, combine the cooled green tea, matcha powder, frozen mango chunks, spinach leaves, avocado, chia seeds, and honey or agave syrup if desired.

If you prefer a colder consistency, add ice cubes to the blender.

Blend the ingredients until smooth and creamy.

Pour into a glass.

NUTRITIONAL INFORMATION

Calories: 200 kcal, Protein: 5g

Fiber: 8g, Fat: 10g

Carbohydrates: 24g

Kiwi Kale Shield Smoothie

INGREDIENTS

1 cup kale, washed and chopped

2 kiwis, peeled and sliced

1/2 banana

1/2 cup pineapple chunks

1 tablespoon chia seeds

1 cup unsweetened almond milk

Ice cubes (optional)

PREPARATION

Place kale, kiwis, banana, pineapple chunks, and chia seeds in a blender.

Add almond milk to the blender.

Blend on high speed.

If desired, add ice cubes and blend again.

Pour the smoothie into a glass.

NUTRITIONAL INFORMATION

Calories: 180 kcal, Protein: 5g

Fiber: 9g, Fat: 3.5g

Carbohydrates: 38g

Orange Carrot Smoothie

INGREDIENTS

1 large carrot, peeled and chopped

1 orange, peeled and segmented

1/2 banana

1/2 cup Greek yogurt (unsweetened)

1 tablespoon flaxseeds

1/2 teaspoon turmeric powder

1 cup water or coconut water

Ice cubes (optional)

PREPARATION

Place chopped carrot, orange segments, banana, Greek yogurt, flaxseeds, and turmeric powder in a blender.

Add water or coconut water to the blender.

Blend on high speed.

If desired, add ice cubes and blend again.

Pour the smoothie into a glass.

NUTRITIONAL INFORMATION

Calories: 220 kcal, Protein: 9g

Fiber: 8g, Fat: 5g

Carbohydrates: 40g

Ginger-Turmeric Citrus Squeeze Smoothie

INGREDIENTS

1 cup mixed citrus fruits (orange, grapefruit, and/or mandarin), peeled and segmented

1/2 banana

1/2 inch fresh ginger, peeled and grated

1/2 teaspoon ground turmeric

1 tablespoon chia seeds

1 cup almond milk (unsweetened)

Ice cubes (optional)

PREPARATION

Place mixed citrus fruits, banana, grated ginger, ground turmeric, and chia seeds in a blender.

Add almond milk to the blender.

Blend on high speed.

If you prefer a colder smoothie, add ice cubes and blend again.

Pour the smoothie into a glass.

NUTRITIONAL INFORMATION

Calories: 220 kcal, Protein: 5g

Fiber: 12g, Fat: 7g

Carbohydrates: 40g

Spirulina Citrus Fortification Smoothie

INGREDIENTS

1 cup fresh orange juice

1/2 banana

1/2 cup pineapple chunks

1 teaspoon spirulina powder

1 tablespoon chia seeds

1 cup spinach leaves (fresh)

Ice cubes (optional)

PREPARATION

In a blender, combine fresh orange juice, banana, pineapple chunks, spirulina powder, chia seeds, and fresh spinach leaves.

Blend on high speed.

If a colder smoothie is desired, add ice cubes and blend again.

Pour the smoothie into a glass.

NUTRITIONAL INFORMATION

Calories: 210 kcal, Protein: 5g

Fiber: 9g, Fat: 3g

Carbohydrates: 45g

Cranberry Cinnamon Smoothie

INGREDIENTS

1/2 cup cranberries (fresh or frozen)

1/2 banana

1/2 cup Greek yogurt

1/2 cup almond milk (unsweetened)

1 teaspoon ground cinnamon

1 tablespoon flaxseeds

1/2 teaspoon honey (optional

Ice cubes (optional)

PREPARATION

In a blender, combine cranberries, banana, Greek yogurt, almond milk, ground cinnamon, flaxseeds, and honey.

Blend on high speed.

If a colder smoothie is desired, add ice cubes and blend again.

Pour the smoothie into a glass.

NUTRITIONAL INFORMATION

Calories: 220 kcal, Protein: 10g

Fiber: 8g, Fat: 7g

Carbohydrates: 32g

Green Tea Berry Smoothie

INGREDIENTS

1 green tea bag

1/2 cup hot water

1/2 cup frozen mixed berries (raspberries, strawberries, blueberries)

1/2 banana

1/2 cup Greek yogurt

1 tablespoon chia seeds

1 teaspoon honey (optional)

Ice cubes (optional)

PREPARATION

Steep the green tea bag in hot water for 3-5 minutes. Allow it to cool.

In a blender, combine the cooled green tea, frozen mixed berries, banana, Greek yogurt, chia seeds, and honey.

Blend on high speed.

If a colder smoothie is desired, add ice cubes and blend again until smooth.

Pour the smoothie into a glass.

NUTRITIONAL INFORMATION

Calories: 220 kcal, Protein: 9g

Fiber: 8g, Fat: 4g

Carbohydrates: 40g

Pineapple Papaya Smoothie

INGREDIENTS

1 cup fresh pineapple chunks

1/2 cup ripe papaya, peeled, seeded, and diced

1 small orange, peeled and segmented

1/2 cup coconut water

1/2 cup plain Greek yogurt

1 tablespoon chia seeds

1 teaspoon turmeric powder

1/2 teaspoon ginger, grated

Ice cubes (optional)

PREPARATION

In a blender, combine the fresh pineapple chunks, diced papaya, orange segments, coconut water, Greek yogurt, chia seeds, turmeric powder, and grated ginger.

Blend on high speed.

If you prefer a colder smoothie, add ice cubes and blend again.

Pour the smoothie into a glass.

NUTRITIONAL INFORMATION

Calories: 250 kcal, Protein: 10g

Fiber: 9g, Fat: 5g

Carbohydrates: 45g

Moringa Mint Smoothie

INGREDIENTS

1 cup fresh spinach leaves

1/2 banana, peeled and sliced

1/2 cup pineapple chunks

1 tablespoon moringa powder

1/4 cup fresh mint leaves

1/2 cup unsweetened almond milk

1/2 cup Greek yogurt

1 tablespoon chia seeds

Ice cubes (optional)

PREPARATION

In a blender, combine fresh spinach leaves, sliced banana, pineapple chunks, moringa powder, fresh mint leaves, almond milk, Greek yogurt, and chia seeds.

Blend on high speed.

If you prefer a colder smoothie, add ice cubes and blend again.

Pour the smoothie into a glass.

NUTRITIONAL INFORMATION

Calories: 220 kcal, Protein: 10g

Fiber: 8g, Fat: 7g

Carbohydrates: 30g

CHAPTER 9: BONUS

Frequently Asked Questions

Why Smoothies for Breast Cancer?

Smoothies offer a convenient and palatable way to incorporate nutrient-dense ingredients into your diet. During breast cancer, when maintaining proper nutrition is crucial, smoothies provide a versatile and enjoyable means to support your overall well-being.

How Can Smoothies Benefit Breast Cancer Patients?

Smoothies can aid in providing essential nutrients, supporting hydration, and addressing potential side effects of cancer treatments. They offer a customizable means to boost immunity, soothe inflammation, and enhance overall nutritional intake.

Can Smoothies Help with Nausea During Treatment?

Yes, certain ingredients like ginger, mint, and hydrating bases can be included in smoothies to help alleviate nausea, a common side effect of cancer treatments. The customizable nature of smoothies allows for the inclusion of ingredients that may be soothing to the digestive system.

Are These Smoothies Suitable for Individuals with Restrictions on Their Diet?

The recipes in this book are designed with adaptability in mind. Whether you have dietary restrictions, allergies, or specific preferences, the variety of ingredients allows for customization to suit individual needs.

How Can Smoothies Help with Weight Management?

For those facing weight loss or challenges with appetite, smoothies can be adjusted for caloric density by incorporating ingredients like nut butter, avocados, or full-fat yogurt. This allows for a concentrated source of energy without compromising nutritional value.

Can I Replace Meals with Smoothies?

Smoothies can be a nutritious addition to your diet but may not replace balanced meals entirely. It is essential to maintain a varied and well-rounded diet to ensure you receive a broad spectrum of nutrients.

What is the Role of Nutrition in Breast Cancer Care?

Nutrition plays a pivotal role in supporting the body during breast cancer treatment. It helps manage side effects, maintain energy levels, and contribute to overall well-being. Understanding the nutritional aspects can empower you to make informed choices.

Are Smoothies a Suitable Option for Everyone?

While smoothies are generally well-tolerated, individual responses may vary. It is advisable to consult with your healthcare providers, especially if you have specific dietary considerations or medical conditions.

Can Smoothies Help with Fatigue?

Nutrient-dense smoothies can provide a source of sustained energy, potentially aiding in managing fatigue during cancer treatments. Ingredients like protein-rich foods and hydrating bases contribute to energy levels.

How Can I Personalize the Recipes to My Taste?

The recipes in this book are crafted with customization in mind. Adjust sweetness levels, experiment with flavor combinations, and tailor the ingredients to suit your taste preferences. The goal is to make your smoothie experience enjoyable and personalized.

Request

Dear Reader,

I have a request. I hope the book **Breast Cancer Smoothies for Beginners** has been helpful in your journey during treatment and recovery. Your opinion means a lot to me and I would appreciate it if you could take a few minutes of your precious time to give your feedback.

Your review will go a long way in helping others with a breast cancer diagnosis or caring for a breast cancer patient make an informed decision about this book.

If you could take a moment, I would be delighted if you could write a review on any book review website such as Amazon, Goodreads, or others. This will assist me in improving my work and also encourage me to continue to create valuable books for you my esteemed reader. I don't take it for granted that you are a part of this journey with me.

Best wishes,

Jane Babb

CONVERSION TABLE

US Standard	Metric
1 teaspoon	5ml
1 tablespoon	15ml
¼ teaspoon	1.25ml
¼ cup	60ml
1/3 cup	75ml
½ cup	125ml
2/3 cup	150ml
¾ cup	175ml
1 cup	250ml

US Standard	Metric
1 cup of Greek yogurt	280g
1 cup of blueberries	190g
1 cup of blackberries	150g
1 cup of strawberries	166g
1 cup of raspberries	125g
1 teaspoon	5g
1 tablespoon	15g

CONCLUSION

Congratulations! As you close the chapter on a journey that extends beyond the realm of recipes, this book isn't just a collection of ingredients; it is a testament to resilience, nourishment, and the transformative power of mindful choices during your breast cancer journey.

As you turn the last page, envision not just the sumptuous smoothies awaiting creation but the empowerment that each sip brings. These recipes are a roadmap to a resilient spirit and a nourished body. From the vibrant hues of antioxidant-rich berries to the comforting warmth of anti-inflammatory spices, each ingredient is carefully chosen to be a companion on your path to healing.

Each recipe is a reminder that wellness is a holistic journey, and every nutrient-rich sip is a step towards vitality. Consistency is the silent hero in the narrative of recovery. As you embrace the importance of consistency, recognize that it extends beyond the kitchen. It's about consistently choosing wellness, consistently acknowledging your strengths, and consistently prioritizing your health. Through this commitment, you lay the foundation for a sustainable and resilient approach to your breast cancer journey.

Through the highs and lows of treatment, the uncertainty of recovery, and the triumphs of resilience, these smoothies stand as a testament to the power of nourishment.

In every swirl of the blender and every refreshing sip, lies the promise of a vibrant tomorrow. Cheers to you, to your health, and to the journey ahead.

All questions and help with recipes should be directed to my email: janebabbnutrition@gmail.com

www.ingramcontent.com/pod-product-compliance
Lightning Source LLC
Chambersburg PA
CBHW071044250726
48653CB00005B/1983